Table of Contents

Introduction

The detox juice diet has become very popular in recent years as an easier way to consume lots of nutrients without having to eat lots of whole fruits and vegetables.

Many people are trying a juice diet for weight loss, overall health, and to overcome a plateau.

A juice detox is a diet that either mainly consists of juicing for a short period of time, or replaces a single meal per day for a longer juice diet.

This book shows various detox recipes juice you can try at home as well as how to make them.

Different Detox Juice to Try

Green Detox Juice

This delicious detox juice makes the perfect meal while on a green juice detox.

Equipment

Juicer

Ingredients

- 2 green apples cut in half
- 3 stalks celery no leaves
- 1 cucumber

- 8 leaves kale

- 1/2 lemon peeled

- 1 piece fresh ginger

- Sprig of mint optional

Instructions

1. Wash all the weight loss juice ingredients well and pat dry.

2. Cut fruit and vegetables into 1-2 inch chunks. Remove any peels.

3. Place all ingredients in a juicer.

4. Process into juice

5. Serve chilled

Tropical Carrot Apple Juice

This is a really delicious drink, and is full of beneficial nutrients such as vitamins, minerals, and antioxidants.

Equipment

Juicer

Ingredients

- 1 large apple quartered
- 1/2 cup pineapple chunks
- 2 large carrots
- 2 pieces fresh ginger

Instructions

1. Wash all the weight loss juice ingredients well and pat dry.

2. Cut fruit and vegetables into 1-2 inch chunks. Remove any peels.

3. Place all ingredients in a juicer.

4. Process into juice

5. Serve chilled

Ginger Zinger

If you're in the market for anti-inflammatory juice, look no further. This ginger-heavy recipe is packed with those antioxidants to help ease any inflammation you've got.

Ingredients

- 2 stalks celery
- ½ cucumber
- 1½ cm ginger
- ½ cup parsley
- ½ lemon
- 1 green apple
- 2 cups spinach

Directions

1. Place all ingredients into your juicer.

2. Serve chilled.

Beet-It-Up

Beets also contain amazing antioxidants, and studies have shown that they can even enhance cognitive function. This juice is perfect before a busy workday!

Ingredients

- 1½ cm fresh ginger

- 3 beets

- 3 carrots

- 3 stalks celery

Directions

1. Place all ingredients into your juicer.

2. Serve chilled.

Kale + Pear

Oh, kale. The queen of trendy greens, the kale in this juice will help you reach your daily veggie quota. Studies have shown that kale juice can even help lower cholesterol!

Ingredients

- 2 stalks kale

- 1 cup spinach

- 1 pear

- ½ lime

- 3 stalks celery

- ½ cucumber

Directions

1. Place all ingredients into your juicer.

2. Serve chilled.

Anti-Inflammatory Tonic

Another anti-inflammatory juice to add to your rotation. This version combines the anti-inflammatory stars—turmeric and ginger—into one nutrient-packed drink.

Ingredients

- 2 cm fresh turmeric
- 4 carrots
- 1 cm fresh ginger
- 1 orange
- ½ lemon
- 3 stalks celery

Directions

1. Place all ingredients into your juicer.

2. Serve chilled.

Electric Green

For an even heavier dose of daily greens, this juice is perfect. With so many vitamins (vitamin C from lime, vitamin A from spinach, and vitamin K from parsley), this juice is a nutritional powerhouse.

Ingredients

- 1 cucumber

- 1 cup parsley

- 1 cup spinach

- 2 green apples

- 2 cm fresh turmeric

- ¾ cucumber

- ½ lime

- 1 green apple

- 2 beets

- 1 cup spinach

Directions

1. Place all ingredients into your juicer.

2. Serve chilled.

Summer Juice

It's always summer with this juice recipe. In addition to the tropical taste, pineapples also offer flavonoids and phenolic acids.

Ingredients

- 1 cup pineapple
- ½ lemon
- 2 carrots
- 2 stalks celery
- 1 cm ginger

Directions

1. Place all ingredients into your juicer.

2. Serve chilled.

Fresh Start

Cilantro is great for keeping your skin clear, while the cucumber is one of the most hydrating vegetables. A fresh start is right—you (and your skin) will stay hydrated all day long.

Ingredients

- 2 stalks celery

- ½ cucumber

- ½ lime

- 1 cup cilantro

- 1 cup kale

- 1 green apple

Directions

1. Place all ingredients into your juicer.

2. Serve chilled.

Carrot Cleanser

Carrots are known for their high vitamin A content, which is great for our eye health. We know how important eye health is to our overall well-being, so add this juice recipe into your morning rotation.

Ingredients

- 4 carrots
- 1 cm fresh ginger
- 1 green apple

Directions

1. Place all ingredients into your juicer.
2. Serve chilled.

Zesty Lemon Apple Juice

This juice for diet is a surprisingly light and tangy detox drink that makes a perfect juice cleanse for breakfast.

Equipment

juicer

Ingredients

- 2 lemons peeled and halved
- 4 apples quartered
- 2 cucumbers halved
- 1 cup water

Instructions

1. Wash all the weight loss juice ingredients well and pat dry.

2. Cut fruit and vegetables into 1-2 inch chunks. Remove any peels.

3. Place all ingredients in a juicer.

4. Process into juice

5. Serve chilled

Kid Friendly Green Juice

If you're looking for a detox juice recipe for kids they will love, this is a good one. The fruits do a good job of masking the taste of the vegetables, and this recipe tastes like a fruit juice.

Equipment

Juicer

Ingredients

- 2 oranges peeled
- 1 lemon peeled
- 1 green apple quartered
- 1 cup baby spinach
- 1 leaf kale

Instructions

1. Wash all the weight loss juice ingredients well and pat dry.
2. Cut fruit and vegetables into 1-2 inch chunks. Remove any peels.
3. Place all ingredients in a juicer.
4. Process into juice and serve chilled

Red Zinger Breakfast Juice

Here's another great juice detox recipe to start your morning with. It's got a great nutritional profile from the vegetables and fruits, and it tastes great, with a slight kick from the lemons.

Equipment

Juicer

Ingredients

- 2 lemons

- 2 carrots

- 2 apples

- 2 beets

Instructions

1. Wash all the weight loss juice ingredients well and pat dry.

2. Cut fruit and vegetables into 1-2 inch chunks. Remove any peels.

3. Place all ingredients in a juicer.

4. Process into juice and serve chilled

Green Spinach Lemonade

This popular detox drink gives you tons of energy, and is really good for you, too. You may want to add a little honey if you like it sweeter, but I would taste it first.

Equipment

Juicer

Ingredients

- 1 cup spinach

- 2 stalks celery

- 4 leaves kale

- 1 piece ginger

- 2 apples

- 1 lemon

Instructions

1. This tart green juice can be made sweeter with another apple, or with a small bit of honey.

2. Wash all the weight loss juice ingredients well and pat dry.

3. Cut fruit and vegetables into 1-2 inch chunks. Remove any peels.

4. Place all ingredients in a juicer.

5. Process into juice and serve chilled

Allergy Fighting Green Detox Juice

If you suffer from seasonal allergies, you should try this delicious detox juice recipe. It has allergy fighting vitamin C rich fruits and vegetables like pineapple, lemon and grapes.

Equipment

Juicer

Ingredients

- 1 cucumber
- 1 cup pineapple
- 1 lemon
- 1 cup seedless grapes
- 1/2 cup parsley
- 1 apple
- 1 mint sprig optional

Instructions

1. Wash all the weight loss juice ingredients well and pat dry.

2. Cut fruit and vegetables into 1-2 inch chunks. Remove any peels.

3. Place all ingredients in a juicer.

4. Process into juice and serve chilled

Orange Dreamsicle Detox Juice

This detox juice is creamy and delicious, just like the old Orange Creamsicle ice cream bars you remember eating when you were a kid. You can even freeze these in popsicle molds for a great frozen treat.

Equipment

Juicer

Ingredients

- 2 medium apples

- 3 stalks celery

- 1 orange peeled

- 2 medium pears

- 1 sweet potato – 5" long cooked and peeled

Instructions

1. Wash all the weight loss juice ingredients well and pat dry.

2. Cut fruit and vegetables into 1-2 inch chunks. Remove any peels.

3. Place all ingredients in a juicer.

4. Process into juice and serve chilled

Easy Start Detox Juice

This makes a good beginner detox juice recipe for those just starting out with juicing, thanks to its simple ingredients and delicious flavors that aren't overwhelming.

Equipment

Juicer

Ingredients

- 2 medium apples

- 3 medium carrots

- 4 celery stalks

Instructions

1. Wash all the weight loss juice ingredients well and pat dry.

2. Cut fruit and vegetables into 1-2 inch chunks. Remove any peels.

3. Place all ingredients in a juicer.

4. Process into juice and serve chilled

Green Ginger Ale Weight Loss Juice

This is my go to recipe, especially when I'm having tummy issues. The taste is amazing, and it's full of nutrients thanks to the variety of ingredients.

Equipment

Juicer

Ingredients

- 3 medium apples

- 2 stalks celery

- 1 cup spinach

- 1 cucumber

- 1 piece ginger root 1" dia

- 1 lime peeled

Instructions

1. Wash all the weight loss juice ingredients well and pat dry.

2. Cut fruit and vegetables into 1-2 inch chunks. Remove any peels.

3. Place all ingredients in a juicer.

4. Process into juice and serve chilled

The "Beets and Treats" detox is rich in beet juice, which helps to clear bile ailments and cleanse away toxicity throughout the blood and liver. The healthier your liver is, the more it can metabolize fat for quick, simple weight loss.

Ingredients

- 178g of beetroot (1 beet)

- 48g or two leaves of cabbage (red)

- 186g (3 medium) carrots

- 46g (1/2 a fruit) lemon

- 136g (1 whole) orange

- 228g (1/4 a fruit) pineapple

- 56g (1 handful) spinach

Directions

1. Simply process all the ingredients together in your favorite blender

2. shake or stir

3. Then serve.

Green Aid" Blitz

Studies have found that eating apples every day not only keeps the doctor away – but helps with weight loss too! Give your digestion system the kick-start that it needs to begin burning away excess fat with a quick and refreshing juice that you can drink all day long.

Ingredients

- 734g (4 medium) apples

- 196g (3 stalks) of celery

- 70g (2 leaves) of kale

- 60g (1 whole lemon - peeled

- 126g (4 cups) of spinach

Directions

1. Chopping your apples, celery, and lemon into chunks.

2. Throw each of those items into your blender, along with your washed kale and celery, and blitz until smooth.

3. Shake up the result, and pour into glasses with a slice of lemon for garnish.

"Any-Time Fat-Loss" Cocktail

The "Any-Time Fat-Loss" cocktail is one of those special blends that works perfectly no matter when you drink it.

Ingredients

- 368g (2 medium) apples

- 84g (2 stalks) of celery

- 306g (1 whole) cucumber

- 182g (5 leaves) of kale

- 46g (1/2 fruit) lemon

- 268g (2 whole) oranges

- 44g (1 handful) of parsley

Directions

1. To mix this juice, chop the parsley and kale together, then dice the apple, cucumber, celery, lemon, and oranges into chunks.

2. Pour the entire ingredient mix into a blender and blitz until smooth.

3. Stir, pour into a glass, and garnish with a
   slice of lemon for that extra-summery look.

BB-USA Green Lemonade Blitz

The "BB-USA Green Lemonade Blitz" combines the
fat-burning power of lemon with the complexion-
boosting radiance of cucumber. In other words –
you won't only lose weight, but your skin will be
glowing too.

Ingredients

- 64g (2 cups) of spinach

- 62g (1 whole) lemon

- 144g (4 leaves) of kale

- 304g (1 whole) cucumber

- 368g (2 medium) apples

Directions

1. Simply dice your apples and cucumber into manageable chunks and throw them into your juicer, along with your lemon, spinach, and kale.

2. Blitz the full mixture until smooth

3. serve in a tall glass with plenty of ice.

Wingman

The celery and orange in your "Wingman" blend will help to maintain a youthful vibrancy in your skin thanks to a healthy dose of vitamin C, while the lemon juice simultaneously battles to burn away fat and cure skin-problems with its inherent antiseptic properties.

Ingredients

- 550g (3 whole) apples
- 196g (3 stalks) of celery
- 154g (1/2 vegetable) cucumber
- 14g (1/2 thumb) of ginger root
- 144g (4 leaves) of kale

- 64g (1 whole) lemon

- 184g (1 whole large) orange - peeled.

Directions

1. Dice the celery, cucumber, lemon, apples, and ginger root into chunks, and throw them into your juices.

2. Add the kale, and blitz the full mixture until smooth.

3. Serve cold.

Beet Nik" Blend (The Ultimate Juice Cleanse)

The "Beet Nik" recipe is particularly beneficial because it replaces a lot of sugary fruits with vitamin-rich vegetables.

Ingredients

- 95g (3 cups) of spinach

- 130g (2 stalks) of celery

- 460g (8 medium) carrots

- 178g (1 whole) beet

- 184g (1 medium) apple

Directions

1. Simply chop all the ingredients into small chunks and add them to your juicer.

2. Blend the mix until smooth

3. Serve cold.

Can't Beet It" Cleanse

The beet juice will cleanse your blood, and your liver, making it easier to metabolize fat, plus you get all the digestion-boosting benefits of carrots, apples, and ginger too!

Ingredients

- 16g (1/2 thumb) of ginger root
- 154g (1/2 vegetable) cucumber
- 196g (3 stalks) of celery
- 246g (4 medium) carrots
- 182 (1 whole) beet
- 368g (2 medium) apples

Directions

1. To blend this mix, simply chop all the ingredients into chunks and pour them into your juicer.

2. Blend until smooth, stir

3. drink instantly

Respect your Roots Healing Blend

This blend comes with carrot juice, which helps to reduce water retention and eliminate excess fluid from the body. Perfect for that quick slim look.

Ingredients

- 178g (1 whole) beetroot
- 614g (10 medium) carrots
- 134g (1 full) sweet potato

Directions

1. Add the ingredients to your juicer in the following order: Beetroot, followed by sweet

potato, followed by a whole lot of diced carrots!

2. Ensure the mixture is smooth

3. Pour into a short glass and enjoy.

The "Morning Glory" Cleanse

If you're feeling lazy and you're in need of a juicing recipe that does a lot for you, without you having to work hard in return – this is your juicing dream come true.

Ingredients

- 178g (1 whole) beetroot

- 126g (2 medium) carrots

- 264g (2 whole) oranges

Directions

1. Chop all three ingredients together and add
   them to your juicer at the same time.

2. Blend until smooth

3. Then serve cold.

The Beautiful "Sunset Blend"

This is probably one of the prettiest juice blends I've ever seen. If you're looking for a way to kick-start your metabolism and add something special to a get-together, then make a batch of these for your friends and family.

Ingredients

- 368g (2 medium) apples
- 178g (1 whole) beetroot
- 74g (1 large) carrot
- 132g (1 whole) orange
- 132g (1 whole) sweet potato

Directions

1. Though this juice mix looks fancy, there's nothing complicated involved in making it. In fact, I usually make a pitcher of this for summer-time garden parties and barbecues.

2. Peel the orange, and carrot and chop them, along with the rest of your ingredients into chunks.

3. Add the full mixture to your juicer and blend until smooth.

The "Red Tangy Spice

The ginger in the "Red Tangy Spice" blend will help to improve your digestion health, eliminate gas, and banish unwanted bloating. The spice will assist in breaking down and digesting fatty foods

Ingredients

- 62g (2 cups) of spinach
- 34g (1/2 fruit) lime
- 15g (1 whole) jalepeno
- 26g (2 stalks) of celery
- 364g (5 large) carrots
- 178g (1 whole) beetroot

Directions

1. Chop the carrots, celery, and beetroot together

2. Add them to your juicer with the whole jalapeno, ginger root, peeled lime, and spinach.

3. Blitz the mixture until smooth and then enjoy the "burn".

Note: If you struggle with spice, de-seed the jalapeno before you add it to the drink.

The "Liver Scrubber"

This combination of beet greens, beet root, and ginger will help to cleanse and detoxify your liver. What's more, the carrots will cleanse the liver and help to aid in faster, more efficient digestion.

Ingredients

- 226g (1 large) apple

- 98g (3 leaves) of beet greens

- 178g (1 whole) beetroot

- 248g (4 medium) carrots

- 66g (1 stalk) of celery

- 14g (1/2 a thumb) of ginger root)

Directions

1. To get the most out of this juice cleanse, slice the ginger root into smaller sections, along with the celery and beet greens.

2. Add those ingredients to your juicer, then dice your apple, carrots, and beetroot.

3. Blend the full mix together until smooth, and serve first thing in the morning.

The "Rock the Beet"

This delicious cleanse generally ends up more like a smoothie than a juice, but you'll still get plenty of fat-fighting benefits, from energy-boosting pears and beetroots, to anti-inflammatory effects.

Ingredients

- 178g (1 whole) beetroot

- 44g (1/2 fruit) lemon

- 536g (3 medium) pears

- 124g (1 cup) rasperries

Directions

1. Peel your lemon, but leave the skin on your pears.

2. Chop the lemon, beetroot, and pears into cubes about the same size as your raspberries

3. Throw the entire mix into your juicer.

4. Blend on full power until smooth, then shake and serve!

The "Heart Beet Cleanse

The "Heart Beet" cleanse is a sweet and fruity way to cleanse your cardiac system and get your metabolic motors running in no time! Carrots have been proven to improve heart health in various studies – lowering cholesterol and reducing your chances of heart disease.

Ingredients

- 192g (1 medium) apple
- 180g (1 whole) beetroot
- 736g (12 medium) carrots
- 48g (1/2 fruit) lemon
- 268g (2 whole) oranges - peeled

Directions

1. Simply peel your orange, and chop it, along with your lemon, carrots, beetroot, and apple into hefty chunks.

2. Throw the lot into your juicer, and hit blend until the mix is smooth.

3. Serve icy cold.

Tropical Mint

This tropical juice will take you right back to the beach, no matter the season. Plus, the mint makes this recipe high in vitamin A, while the lemon adds some vitamin C to the mix.

Ingredients

- 2 stalks celery

- ½ cucumber

- 2 cups spinach

- 3 cups mint leaves

- 1 cup pineapple

- ½ lemon

Directions

1. Place all ingredients into your juicer.

2. Serve chilled.

Iron Boost

You can juice broccoli. In fact, the vegetable has quite a lot of iron, making this juice the perfect recipe to raise your iron levels.

Ingredients

- ½ cucumber

- 2 stalks celery

- 1 cup romaine lettuce

- 1 cup broccoli

- 1 green apple

- ½ lime

Directions

1. Place all ingredients into your juicer.

2. Serve chilled.

Sweet Beet

For those of you who want the antioxidant properties of beets but aren't into the strong taste, this version offers the same nutritious benefits with a more subtle beet flavor.

Ingredients

*   1 beet

*   2 carrots

- 3 stalks celery

- ½ lemon

- 1 cm ginger

- 1 green apple

Directions

1. Place all ingredients into your juicer.

2. Serve chilled.